Amene FKI
Mounira HAJJAJI
Kaouthar JMAL

Occupational dermatoses in instrumentalists

Amene FKI
Mounira HAJJAJI
Kaouthar JMAL

Occupational dermatoses in instrumentalists

ScienciaScripts

Imprint

Any brand names and product names mentioned in this book are subject to trademark, brand or patent protection and are trademarks or registered trademarks of their respective holders. The use of brand names, product names, common names, trade names, product descriptions etc. even without a particular marking in this work is in no way to be construed to mean that such names may be regarded as unrestricted in respect of trademark and brand protection legislation and could thus be used by anyone.

Cover image: www.ingimage.com

This book is a translation from the original published under ISBN 978-620-6-72369-1.

Publisher:
Sciencia Scripts
is a trademark of
Dodo Books Indian Ocean Ltd. and OmniScriptum S.R.L publishing group

120 High Road, East Finchley, London, N2 9ED, United Kingdom
Str. Armeneasca 28/1, office 1, Chisinau MD-2012, Republic of Moldova, Europe
Printed at: see last page
ISBN: 978-620-3-28583-3

Contents

1 INTRODUCTION

For several years now, the fight against infection has been a public health priority. Many professional sectors, particularly the healthcare sector, have had to comply with strict hygiene standards, which has led to an intensification of disinfection procedures and the consequent massive use of disinfectant products (1).

A disinfectant is a product that eliminates microbes present in an inert solid or liquid medium. This operation is called disinfection (2).

These products are used for disinfecting premises (surfaces, floors and atmosphere) and medical equipment (soaking disinfection of medical instruments, machine disinfection of optical exploration systems, disinfection of dialysis circuits, bedpans, hospital waste skips, etc.). The aim is to limit as far as possible the risk of cross-transmission of germs between patients, and therefore to limit nosocomial infections (2,3).

The main components found in these products are: aldehydes, quaternary ammoniums, alcohols, oxidants, phenolic derivatives, biguanides, diamides and carbanilides. In addition, the dermatological risk varies depending on the type of exposure and the physicochemical characteristics of the products (2,4).

Most of these products are corrosive and sensitising, and can cause disabling occupational skin conditions in exposed workers. Dermatoses caused by disinfectants can have a variety of clinical manifestations, but the main forms are irritant dermatitis, allergic contact dermatitis, contact urticaria, decompensations of atopic dermatitis and a few rarer forms such as photosensitivity reactions, polymorphic erythema and generalized eruptions (2,3).

In this context, we wanted to take a closer look at occupational dermatoses found in employees exposed to disinfectants in the workplace. To this end, we carried out a cross-sectional descriptive study among instrument technicians in the operating theatre of the Habib Bourguiba University Hospital in Sfax and in the gynaecology unit of the Hedi Chaker University Hospital in Sfax, Tunisia. The objectives of this study were to detect occupational dermatoses in instrument technicians, to assess the chemical risk associated with the use of

disinfectants in operating theatres and to propose appropriate preventive measures.

1 Type of study :

This study is a descriptive cross-sectional survey conducted in the operating theatre of the Habib Bourguiba University Hospital in Sfax and the gynaecology unit of the Hedi Chaker University Hospital in Sfax, Tunisia, over a period of 2 months.

2 Population studied :

The population studied was made up of instrument technicians assigned to the operating theatre of the Habib Bourguiba University Hospital, as well as the Gynecology department of the Hedi Chaker University Hospital.

Before the start of the survey, and during an individual interview, each member of staff was informed of the objectives of the survey and of his or her right to refuse to take part in the study and/or to withdraw without having to provide any justification.

2.1 Inclusion criteria :

We included all the instrumentalists who performed the disinfection task as part of their hospital activity and who were present during the site visits carried out during the study period and who agreed to take part in the survey.

2.2 Exclusion criteria :

We excluded staff who did not handle disinfectants and subjects who did not consent to take part in the study.

3 Assessment tools :

3.1 Self-questionnaire (appendix 1):

We carried out a self-administered questionnaire which collected the following data:

3.1.1 Socio-demographic and occupational characteristics:

In this section, we collected information on age, sex, department, grade, length of service, working hours and number of hours worked per day. We also asked participants whether they had any extra-curricular activities (housework, gardening, DIY....).

3.1.2 Medical history :

We recorded the pathological antecedents of our study population, in particular dermatological antecedents (urticaria, eczema, irritant dermatitis, etc.), personal and/or family atopy (asthma, rhinoconjunctivitis, atopic dermatitis) and respiratory antecedents (rhinitis, asthma, etc.).

3.1.3 Screening for occupational dermatoses :

We asked the participants about any current or past skin lesions on their hands that had occurred at any time during their professional activity. The hands were then clinically examined for skin lesions.

The diagnosis of allergic contact dermatitis (ACD) was suspected in the presence of erythematous, oozing, pruritic lesions with a crumbly outline extending beyond the contact area. In its chronic phase, CAD was suspected in the presence of lichenified, fissured and pigmented skin with new episodes of vesiculation, oozing and crusts occurring due to new exposure to the allergen (5).

The diagnosis of irritant contact dermatitis (ICD) was suspected in the presence of macular or papular lesions with an erythematous appearance, erythemato-redematous or erythematosquamous lesions that appeared rapidly and did not extend beyond the areas of contact with the irritant agent, with a sensation of stinging or burning (acute CID), or other features suggestive of chronic CID (cutaneous dryness, erythematosquamous dermatitis, reactive hyperkeratosis, cracks, disappearance of fingerprints) (5).

We then asked the subjects who had presented these skin lesions on the hand if they had benefited from any investigations (patch test, prick test, other specific tests (open test; roat test; use test), CBC, total IgE, specific IgE), as well as about any treatment received and subsequent outcome.

We accepted the occupational origin of the dermatosis according to the Mathias criteria (6).

The diagnosis was made when at least four of these seven criteria were positive (Table I).

Table I: Mathias criteria for the diagnosis of contact dermatitis

occupational

- Appearance of lesions and history consistent with contact dermatitis

- Occupational exposure to irritants or allergens

- Anatomical distribution compatible with the stain and 1 exposure

- Temporal relationship between exposure and onset of dermatitis compatible with an occupational origin

- Non-occupational exposure excluded

- Improvement when exposure is stopped

- Confirmation of occupational origin by additional tests.

3.1.4 Extracutaneous disorders :

Signs of extracutaneous damage were investigated, including respiratory damage (allergic rhinitis, asthma, respiratory irritation) and eye damage (allergic or irritative conjunctivitis).

3.2 Assessment of the chemical risk associated with the use of disinfectants:

We carried out an assessment of the chemical risk of disinfectants in the operating theatre of the Habib Bourguiba University Hospital and the gynaecology ward of the Hedi Chaker University Hospital, using an occupational risk assessment guide (7).

Applying this guide enabled us to identify the hazardous situations associated with each disinfectant product, to estimate for each hazardous situation: the severity of the potential damage and the frequency with which employees are exposed to the hazards, and to conclude that action should be prioritised on the basis of these last two parameters.

This method is divided into five stages:

1- Drawing up a global inventory of disinfectant products handled in the operating theatre

2- Identify the hazardous situations associated with each product, by checking safety data sheets and conditions of use, systematically examining workplaces and observing disinfection processes and procedures.

3- Estimate for each hazardous situation: the severity of the potential damage, the level of exposure of workers to the hazards (Table II), and the level of protection (Table III).

4- Ranking risks:

Risk ranking was used to determine the priorities for the action plan, and is based on the severity of the potential damage and the level of exposure of employees to the hazards (Figure 1).

5- Propose appropriate prevention and protection measures while respecting the general principles of prevention (7) :

- Eliminate hazards or dangerous situations,

- Controlling risks through collective measures,

- Propose the repositioning or acquisition of new personal protective equipment.

All this data is stored on a form (Table IV).

Table II: Estimated severity and level of exposure to hazards

The severity of potential damage		
1.	Low	Accident or illness without time off work
2.	Average	Accident or illness with time off work
3.	Grave	Accident or illness with partial permanent disability
4.	Very serious	Fatal accident or illness

The level of exposure of employees to hazards

1.	Low	Exposure on the order of once a year
2.	Average	Exposure on the order of once a month
3.	Frequente	Exposure on the order of once a week
4.	very Frequente	Daily or permanent exhibition

NB: The severity is estimated on the basis of the work situation and the statistics of the incidents and accidents.

Table III: Level of protection

Level of protection	*Denomination*
1	Collective protection
2	Personal protective equipment or prevention instructions
3	No protection

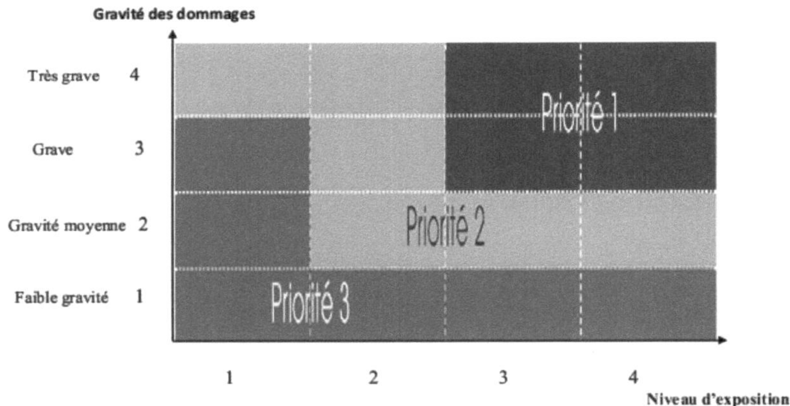

Figure 1: Risk hierarchy

Table IV: Model summary table

Disinfectant	Dangerous situations	Potential damage	Risk		Level of protection	Priority level	Proposed prevention measures
			Gravite	Frequency			

4   Statistical analysis :

The data was entered and processed using the 20eme version of SPSS (Statistical Package for the Social Sciences).

We carried out a descriptive study to record all the characteristics of the population studied and any skin disorders. Quantitative variables were described using means and standard deviations. Qualitative variables were described using proportions.

5 Bibliographic research :

The bibliographic search was carried out using the following search engines: science direct.com, em-consulte.com and pubmed.com, using the following key words: disinfectants, occupational dermatosis, healthcare staff, operating theatre.

6 Ethical considerations :

The anonymity of the study subjects was respected. The study was conducted with strict respect for medical confidentiality and the consent of the individuals involved, with no conflict of interest. Occupational risk assessment was carried out by means of a site visit following administrative approval.

3 RESULTS

1   Socio-professional characteristics:

Forty-five instrumentalists took part in the survey, representing a participation rate of 71.4%.

1.1 Age :

The average age of the participants was 39.7 +/- 10.3 years, with extremes ranging from 26 to 59 years.

1.2 Gender :

More than half the participants were female, with a sex ratio of 0.66 (Figure 2).

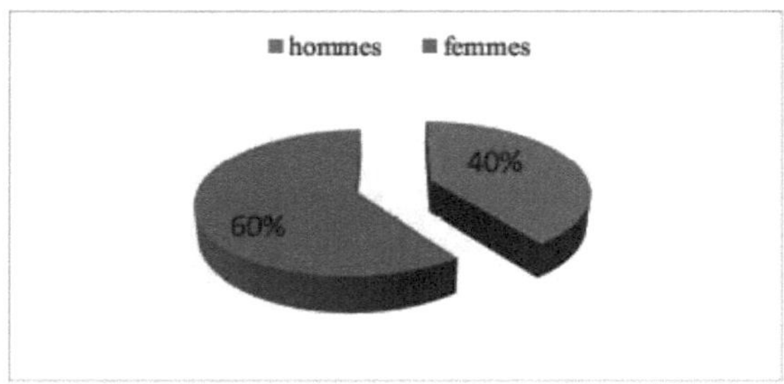

Figure 2: Breakdown of the study population by gender

1.3 Professional grade

Almost two-thirds of the participants were senior operating instrumentation technicians (Figure 3).

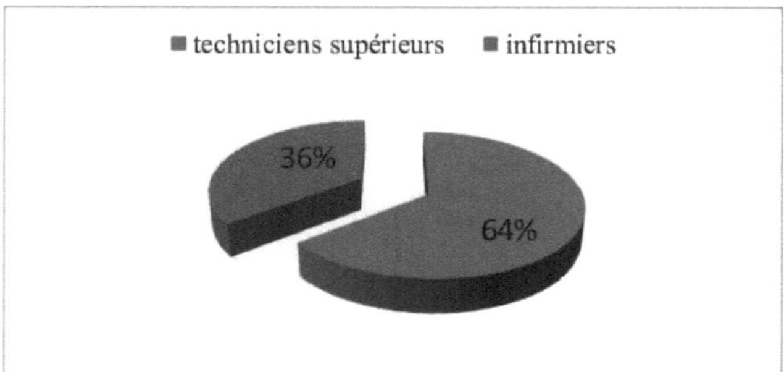

Figure 3: Distribution of the study population according to grade

1.4 Department :

The instrumentalists in our study population were concentrated in the operating theatres of the

Habib Bourguiba University Hospital (n=39) and the gynaecology operating theatre of the

Hedi Chaker University Hospital (n=6) (Table V).

Table V: Breakdown of the study population by operating theatre of assignment

Operating theatre	Workforce	Percentage
General surgery	10	22,2
Orthopaedics	11	24,4
Gynecology	6	13,3
Ear, nose and throat	4	8,9
Neurosurgery	4	8,9
Urology	3	6,7
Cardiovascular	3	6,7
maxillofacial	2	4,4
Ophthalmology	2	4,4
Total	45	100

1.5 Previous professional experience :

The average working life was 14.2 ± 10.8 years (ranging from 6 months to 38 years) (Figure

4).

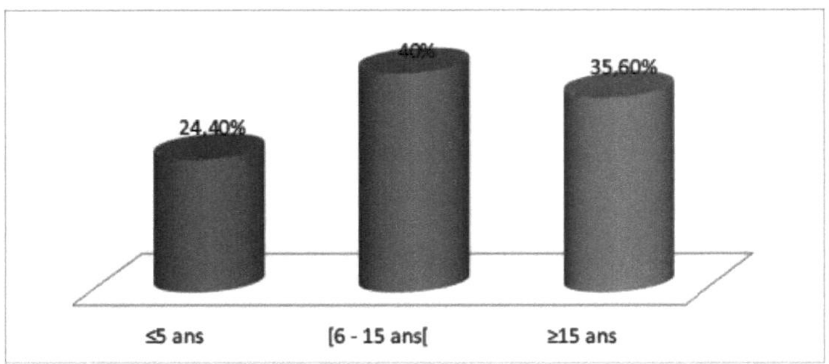

Figure 4: Breakdown by length of service

1.6 Work schedule :

Most instrumentalists (68.9%) worked variable hours (Figure 5). Night work concerned 41%

of those questioned, including 5 cases of fixed night work.

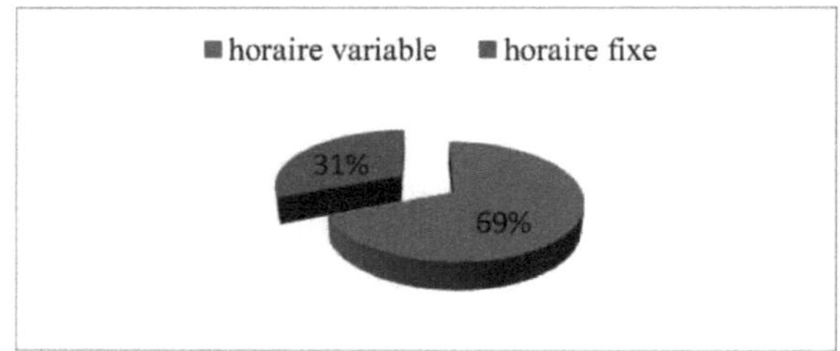

Figure 5: Breakdown by working hours

1.7 Extra-curricular activities

More than half of the study population (60%) did not have an extra-professional activity

(table VI).

Table VI: Breakdown according to the presence of an extra-curricular activity

Extra-curricular activities	Workforce	%
Nothing	27	60
Housework	13	28,9
Sport	4	8,9

2 Medical history :

2.1 Dermatological history :

When we asked the instrumentalists about their dermatological antecedents for which they

had received medical treatment, we found that 10 cases had consulted a doctor for skin

problems. Most of these cases were irritant dermatitis (Table VII).

Table VII: Breakdown by dermatological antecedents

Dermatological history	Workforce	%
Irritant dermatitis	5	11,1
Onychomycosis	2	4,4
Hand eczema	1	2,2
Psoriasis	1	2,2
Demodecie	1	2,2
Total	10	22,1

2.2 History of atopy :

A history of personal atopy was reported by 15.7% (n=7) of the instrumentalists, with allergic

rhinoconjunctivitis in all cases.

A history of family atopy was reported by 22.2% of the staff questioned, in the form of

allergic rhinitis (5 cases), asthma (3 cases) and atopic dermatitis (1 case).

2.3 Respiratory history:

A history of allergic rhinitis was noted in 46.7% of cases, asthma in 11.1% and respiratory

irritation in 1 case.

2.4 Other medical history :

Other antecedents were found in 28.9% of instrumentalists (table VIII).

Table VIII: Breakdown by other medical history

Other antecedents	Workforce	%
Low back pain	5	11,1
HTA	3	6,7
Carpal tunnel syndrome	2	4,4
Hypothyroidism	1	2,2
Shoulder tendonitis	1	2,2
Synovitis of the hand	1	2,2
Gonarthrosis	1	2,2

3   Screening for occupational dermatoses :

3.1 Screening for new cases of contact dermatitis:

By carrying out a detailed interview and clinical examination of the lesions present on the day of the survey, we detected 8 new cases of contact dermatitis of the ICD (5 cases), CDD (1 case) and urticaria (2 cases) type (Figure 6).

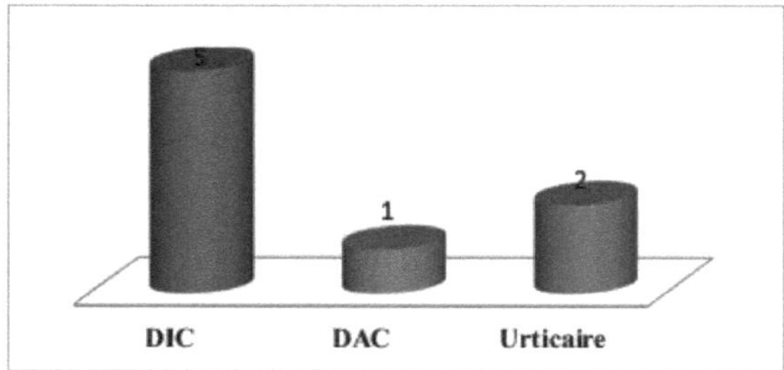

Figure 6: New cases of contact dermatitis in instrumentalists

3.2 Screening for occupational origin using Mathias' criteria

According to Mathias' criteria, the diagnosis of occupational dermatosis was retained in 31.1% of instrumentalists. These dermatoses were irritant contact dermatitis (10 cases), allergic contact dermatitis (2 cases) and urticaria (2 cases) (Figure 7).

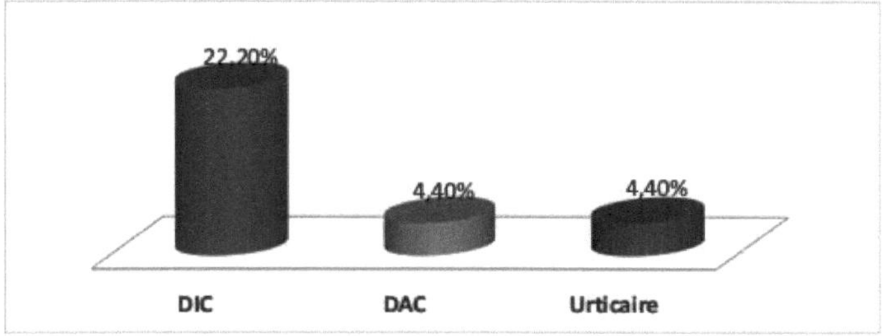

Figure 7:   Occupational dermatitis in instrumentalists

The time from onset of these dermatoses to recruitment ranged from 3 months to 30 years, with an average of 6.7 years.

7.3 Additional examinations

None of the patients had their contact dermatitis investigated, either because they had not been consulted or because of a lack of allergological tests.

7.4 Therapeutic management :

Patients with CID had been treated with reparative creams in 2 cases and moisturisers in 2 others. One patient with CAD had received a dermocorticoid-based treatment.

7.5 Evolution :

The course was marked by persistence of the dermatosis in 5 cases, healing in 1 case and recurrence in 10 cases (Figure 8).

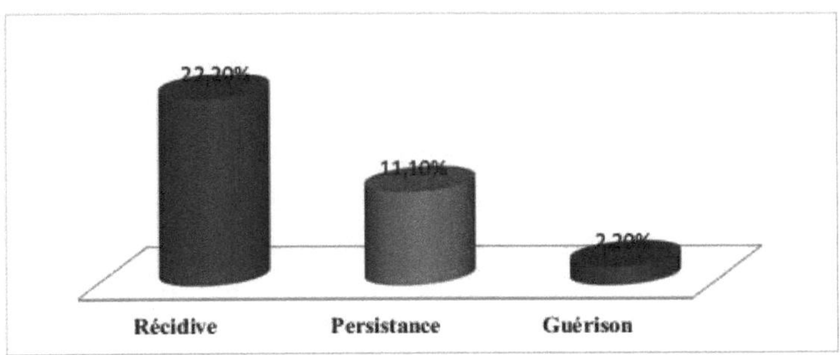

4 Extra-cutaneous disorders associated with the use of disinfectants :

4.1 Respiratory disorders :

More than half of the instrumentalists (55.6%) had signs of rhinitis, 40% of which were attributed to the use of disinfectants in their work.

Symptoms suggestive of a respiratory gene related to the handling of disinfectants were found in 7 instrumentalists. One case of latex-induced asthma was reported (Figure 9).

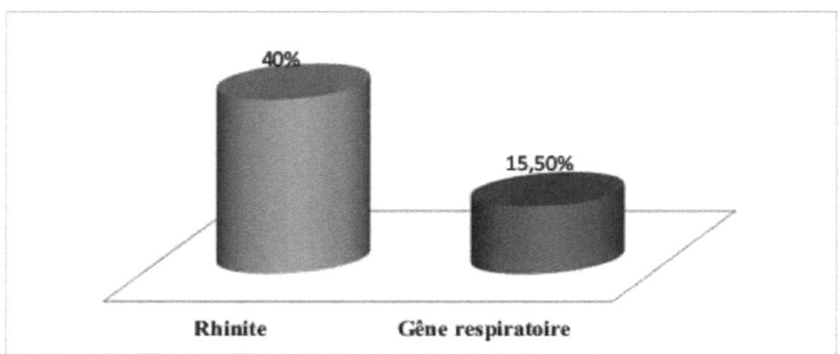

Figure 9:   Breakdown of respiratory problems related to disinfectants

4.2 Eye damage :

Allergic and/or irritative conjunctivitis was reported by 9 instrumentalists (20%).

5   Medical and legal follow-up:

Patients with persistent or recurrent skin lesions were referred to the Dermatology Department for confirmation of the diagnosis and medical follow-up.

Similarly, staff with respiratory symptoms were referred to the Pneumology Department for investigation, diagnostic confirmation and treatment.

From a professional point of view, all the instrumentalists suffering from occupational dermatitis kept the same workstation, subject to the application of appropriate preventive measures depending on the nature of the disinfectant products handled.

With regard to the declaration of an occupational disease, given the unavailability of epicutaneous tests at the time of the survey, we were unable to confirm the etiological agent and therefore to declare CAD. However, in the case of latex-induced asthma, a declaration under table 44 bis of occupational diseases was recommended.

6 Assessment of the chemical risk associated with the use of disinfectants in operating theatres:

6.1 Inventory of disinfectants used :

The most commonly used disinfectants were hexanios (75.5%), Cidex (40%) and formaldehyde (31.1%) (Table IX).

Table IX: Breakdown by disinfectants used

Disinfectants	Active ingredients	Workforce %	
Hexanios G+R	Quaternary ammoniums, Biguanide	34	75,5
Cidex	Glutaraldhehyde	18	40
Formaldehyde	Formaldehyde	14	31,1
DDN9 (Neutral disinfectant detergent)	Didecylmethylammonium propionate	13	29,9
Anios special DJP	Chloride didecyldimethylammonium chloride, hydrochloride polyhexamethylene biguanide	11	24,4
Aseptanios Terminal HPH	Formaldehyde, N-3-aminopropyl N-dodecylpropane1,3-diamine, ethanol.	5	11,1
Bleach	sodium hypochlorite	5	11,1
Nosocomia	Quaternary ammonium Biguanide, isopropanol	4	8,9
Surfanios	Quaternary ammonium, amino acid	2	4,4

6.2 Assessment of instrumentalists' knowledge of modalities on the use of disinfectants and their possible health effects :

A lack of training in the procedures and rules for using disinfectants concerned 51.1% of the instrumentalists questioned.

Only 37.8% of staff were aware of the health risks of disinfectants.

6.3 Hierarchisation of the chemical risks of disinfectant products:

Our approach to chemical risk assessment enabled us to collect all the data specific to each disinfectant product in summary tables, using the method described above.

The data collected is summarised in the occupational risk hierarchy tables (table X and its sequels).

Table X: Hierarchisation of the chemical risk of disinfectants

Disinfectants	Dangerous situations	Potential damage	Risk		Level of protection	Priority level	Proposed prevention measures
			Gravite	Frequency			
Hexanios G+R	- Handling in confined and unconfined spaces aeres, without port of means of protection suitable individuals	- Skin corrosion / skin irritation - Eye lesions severe / irritation ocular	2	4	3	2	- Good ventilation of premises - Use appropriate PPE (waterproof gloves, etc.). in neoprene complying with standard NF EN374, safety goggles with side protection, in In case of insufficient ventilation, wear a appropriate breathing apparatus (mask filtering organic vapours - type A protection))
Cidex	Handling	Eye/	2	4	3	2	- Adequate ventilation

Cidex in confined, non-ventilated spaces without wearing adequate personal protective equipment	respiratory/ skin irritation Skin allergy Respiratory allergy		- Suction at source - Use appropriate PPE (safety goggles, nitrile or butyl rubber gloves, neoprene, filtering breathing apparatus) - Store in a cool, well-ventilated place away from sources of heat.

Table X: Hierarchisation of the chemical risk of disinfectants (cont. 1)

Products Dangerous situations for disinfectants Any	Damage	Risk Level of Level of " .. , ..., Gravity Frequency protection priority	Proposed prevention measures
- skin burns - eye lesions „ . , ᵣ . serious. -Handling formalin■ „ " . skin irritation in confined spaces and . .. x , _ skin allergy **Formol** not aerated, without wearing °. , / .. - irritation means of protection . ■ j- -j и ᴊ-x breathing mdividual ... ⁿ - anomalies genetics - cancer			- Substitution of formalin by another disinfectant product - Handling formalin in an air-conditioned room under a fume hood - Use suitable PPE (respiratory **44** respiratory equipment fitted with anti-gas filter(s) and **3** vapours (combined filters) in compliance with the standard NF EN14387, goggles complying with standard NF EN166, waterproof gloves complying with standard NF EN374, appropriate protective clothing)
„ ... skin burn - Handling without wearing ,			-Ensure adequate ventilation -Use appropriate PPE (safety goggles, safety glasses, etc.)

-skin irritation | | | | 242 | side protection complying with NF

NMS9 means of protection, | . | | | 3 | EN166, gloves resistant to

. j. .j и „„ₓ -eye lesions | | | | chemical in accordance with standard NF EN374).

ⁿ   serious

Table X: Hierarchisation of the chemical risk of disinfectants (continued 2)

Products Dangerous disinfectants situations	Damage Any	Risk		Level of protection	Level of priority	Proposed prevention measures
		Gravite	Frequence			
DJP	-Exposure to the product by inhalation and skin contact	- burn /skin irritation e - serious eye damage - respiratory irritation	2	3	3	2	- Do not allow access to the room during disinfection. - Use appropriate PPE (safety goggles complying with standard NF EN166, chemical-resistant gloves complying with standard NF EN374, breathing apparatus....).
HPH	- Unsafe handling without wearing adequate personal protective equipment	- serious eye damage. - skin irritation - skin allergy - respiratory irritation - genetic abnormalities - cancer	4	3	3	1	- Substitution with another disinfectant product - Adequate ventilation - Use appropriate PPE (breathing apparatus fitted with anti-gas and vapour filter(s) (Combination filters) in accordance with standard NF EN14387, side protection goggles in accordance with standard NF EN166, waterproof gloves in accordance with standard NF

EN374, appropriate

protective clothing).

Table X: Hierarchisation of the chemical risk of disinfectants (continued 3)

Products disinfectants	Dangerous situations	Damage Any	Risk		Level of protection	Level of priority	Proposed prevention measures
			Gravite	Frequence			
Nosocomia, surfanios							- Good ventilation of premises - Use suitable PPE (waterproof neoprene gloves complying with standard NF EN374, safety goggles with side protection, in the event of insufficient ventilation, wear suitable respiratory equipment (mask filtering organic vapours - type A protection)).
	- Handling in confined and non-ventilated spaces without wearing adequate personal protective equipment	- Skin corrosion - skin irritation - Serious eye damage -eye irritation	2	4	3	2	
Bleach	-Unsafe handling, without wearing adequate personal protective equipment	-skin burns -serious eye damage. - skin irritation. - Irritation of the respiratory tract.	1	3	3	3	- Do not mix with other products, particularly acids. - use appropriate PPE (safety goggles complying with standard NF EN166, appropriate protective gloves resistant to chemical agents complying with standard NF EN374 in natural latex - PVC - Nitrile or Neoprene rubber, etc.).

4 DISCUSSION

It is true that over the last few years, disinfection tasks in the healthcare sector have been stepped up to meet strict hygiene standards, leading to massive use of disinfectants. On the other hand, this has increased workers' exposure to products that are, for the most part, corrosive and/or sensitising, which explains the high incidence of occupational dermatitis in this sector. In addition, employees are often poorly informed about the nature of the products they use and the protective measures required when handling them. Improper use of these products (8) and inadequate protective equipment (9,10) increase the risk of these employees developing skin lesions.

1 Strengths and limitations of the study :

Our study is characterised by certain strong points that deserve to be mentioned. It is a cross-sectional descriptive study with two main objectives: to screen for occupational dermatoses in a population of workers exposed to disinfectants, and to assess the chemical risks associated with the use of disinfectants in operating theatres. These two objectives are of major interest, given that screening is one of the aspects of occupational medicine that promotes the health of workers, and that risk assessment is considered to be the first step in an effective prevention approach that can be of great benefit to the community, Screening for the toxicological effects of these products, most of which are unknown and underestimated, makes it possible to identify the most frequent risks and to adopt a more effective prevention strategy, while ensuring that the various players involved adhere to the proposed measures. Our approach therefore focused on work habits and procedures for using disinfectants, in order to encourage behaviour more conducive to maintaining the well-being of these workers, and to teach them the rules of safe handling by proposing preventive measures appropriate to each situation.

Despite the strengths of our study, certain limitations should be mentioned. The size of our study is small, which limits the interpretation we can make of the results. In addition, the occupational dermatoses detected in our study population may be the consequence of several occupational exposures in operating theatres other than disinfectants (latex gloves, nickel, working in a humid environment, etc.) and it is therefore difficult to confirm the etiological agents of these dermatoses, especially as allergological tests were not available at the time of the study. It should also be remembered that the diagnosis of occupational dermatoses is always difficult. Firstly, in terms of the clinical type of dermatitis, the distinction between irritant dermatitis and allergic contact eczema is not always clear, but also in terms of identifying the causative agent in the workplace.

In addition, the control and use of the chemical risk assessment tool adopted in our study should take account of the complexities of the method, which lie in the fact that risk control actions apply to several types of situation, with general interventions adapted to all risks and others that are more specific.

2   Occupational dermatoses :

2.1 Prevalence :

The prevalence of occupational dermatoses in our study population was estimated at 31.1%. Numerous studies confirm the high risk of occupational dermatitis in the healthcare sector, with a prevalence of around 20-30% (11,12). In Italy, hospital staff constitute the 5eme group at risk of hand eczema (12). Similarly, in a study carried out in the Ile de France region (13), based on an occupational dermatology consultation, the healthcare sector was the most frequent source of occupational dermatoses (24%).

Nurses are frequently affected; the incidence was 14.5 cases per 100 person-years according to the prospective study by Smit et al. in 1994 (14). In the UK (15), the incidence is estimated at 136.9 per million (Epiderm network report 2002-2005). In Northern Bavaria, Mahler et al (16) analysed cases of occupational dermatoses recorded between 1990 and 1999. They reported an annual incidence of 7.3 per 10,000 healthcare workers In a recent study in Denmark, the prevalence of hand eczema in healthcare workers (n = 3181 with a response rate of 71%) was twice as high as in the general population (17). In the questionnaire study,

Flyvholm et al. (18) report the prevalence of self-reported hand eczema by profession: student nurses (32.1%), nurses (29.7%), care assistants (27.1%), cleaning staff (19.1%); laboratory technicians (16.9%), secretaries (16.5%), doctors (15.8%), administrative staff (12.3%), physiotherapists and occupational therapists (7.9%).

As far as the agents involved are concerned, disinfectants, along with gloves, are the main causes of contact dermatitis in healthcare workers (12,19).

2.2 Clinical forms of occupational dermatoses :

2.2.1 Irritant contact dermatitis (ICD) :

ICD was the most frequent clinical form (22.2% of instrumentalists included in our study). This finding was consistent with several international studies (20-23) which have shown that CID is more common than CAD in healthcare workers. In fact, in the study by Paul et al (24), CID was the most common clinical form in healthcare workers (43.6%). Similarly, Higgins et al (25) found that CID was the most frequent form in healthcare workers followed up for occupational dermatoses (79.1%).

However, several authors have reported higher rates of CAD than CID in healthcare workers (26-29), but in these latter studies, the rates varied with occupational subgroups and the dermatosis was not always work-related.

This frequency of ICDs in this sector of activity, and particularly among the instrumentalists in our study, can be explained by the fact that these employees regularly use disinfectant products during disinfection procedures. Most of these products are highly irritant and are therefore probably largely responsible for the appearance of irritative lesions in these subjects. However, it should be pointed out that there are many co-factors of irritation in this sector of activity (2): chemical factors, of course, in particular professional soaps and industrial detergents, which increase the permeability of the skin by creating a dysfunction in the cutaneous barrier (3) and which, according to Dickel et al, the leading cause of occupational skin irritation (30), but also mechanical factors (intensive and repeated hand washing (31)) and finally physical factors (working in a damp environment, the occlusive effect of protective gloves and exposure to cold (32)).

2.2.2 Allergic contact dermatitis (ACD) :

Two instrumentalists (4.4%) included in our study had CAD, i.e. a rate of 14.2% of all occupational dermatoses found. This rate is lower than that reported in the literature and may be related to the small size of the study population. Paul et al (24) reported a rate of 25.6% of DAC and 20.5% of irritant dermatitis associated with allergic contact dermatitis among care workers followed up in an occupational dermatology consultation.

Similarly, Higgins et al (25) reported a 49.7% rate of CAD among 555 healthcare workers followed up in an occupational dermatology clinic in Australia over a 22-year period.

In the study by Gargon-Michel (13) of 145 cases of occupational dermatoses in all sectors, CAD was more common than ICD (41% versus 26%), with an association between CAD and ICD reported in 9% of cases.

2.2.3 Contact urticaria :

Contact urticaria was noted in 2 cases and was most likely linked to an allergy to the latex proteins contained in the gloves.

In the study conducted by Higgins (25), skin allergy to latex gloves accounted for 13% of occupational dermatitis in healthcare workers.

Although the most frequent causes of immediate allergic reactions are latex proteins in care and cleaning staff, certain antiseptics or disinfectants can also cause contact urticaria (chlorhexidine, polyvidone-iodine, formaldehyde, chloramine). Immediate allergy to chlorhexidine is mediated by IgE: it can be severe with anaphylactic reactions, mainly following mucosal or parental exposure (33). More than 30 cases of anaphylactic shock have been reported, mostly by Japanese authors. In Japan, the use of chlorhexidine gluconate on mucous membranes has been banned since 1984 (33-35).

3   Extracutaneous damage caused by the use of disinfectants:

Signs of rhinitis attributed to the use of disinfectants were found in 40% of instrumentalists. Symptoms suggestive of a respiratory gene related to the handling of disinfectants were found in 7 instrumentalists. Signs of conjunctivitis were reported by 9 instrumentalists (20%).

In France, the National Observatory of Occupational Asthma (ONAP) ranked the health sector second in the 1996-1998 survey, after bakers and confectioners (36), and considered disinfectants used in medical environments, along with latex, to be the most frequent causes of occupational asthma (36). Similarly, the National Institute for Occupational Safety and Health (NIOCH) reported an asthma prevalence of 8% in hospitals (37).

In the literature, more than 40 articles have documented an association between cleaning products, and more specifically disinfectants used in hospitals, and asthma (38-42). In fact, six disinfectants meet the AOEC (Association of Occupational and Environmental Clinics) criteria for substances classified as causing asthma (43).

The diagnosis of disinfectant-induced asthma should be made in the presence of rhinitis or asthma, chronologically linked to work, in a person exposed to disinfectants at work. Symptoms appear after several months (44,45) or years (46) of exposure, and sometimes after only a few weeks (45).

Allergic rhinitis associating nasal pruritus, sneezing, aqueous rhinorrhea and nasal obstruction is often the first clinical manifestation of respiratory allergy (45,47). It may be accompanied by conjunctivitis (48), manifested by conjunctival pruritus and lacrimation. Oculonasal symptoms begin within minutes of sensitising contact (49). Elsewhere, there are signs of irritation of the mucous membranes associated with a sensation of oculonasal burning (50,51). Asthma occurs at the same time as rhinitis (49), or complicates it after several months or years, or is the first manifestation of respiratory disease (51). The asthma may be old, atopic, a- or pauci-symptomatic, or recently reactive [9, 24], raising the question of the irritant rather than sensitising role of the biocides present (45). In other cases, the onset of asthma has followed accidental exposure, and a diagnosis of irritant-induced asthma may be wrongly made (52).

4 Assessment of the chemical risk associated with the use of disinfectants in

operating theatres:

Assessment of the chemical risk associated with the use of disinfectants in operating theatres has enabled us to establish preventive priorities and implement a strategy to improve control of this chemical risk.

Assessing chemical risk is often difficult because of the large number of chemical agents and preparations used, but also because of the lack of knowledge about the hazards involved. Worldwide, almost 18 million organic and inorganic chemical structures have been registered in the *Chemical Abstract Service* published in 2001 by the *American Chemical Society*. The number of substances for which partial toxicological information is available is only ﹍50,000, according to the NIOSH *Registry of Toxic Effects of Chemical Substances* (RTECS) database in the USA. According to the US *National Library of Medicine* database, the number of hazardous substances for which valid data are available is around 4,500 (53). This difficulty in understanding chemical risk is even more critical for small establishments where the activity requires the use of chemicals (54). In this context, various approaches have been developed in Europe by research bodies and companies. In the early 1990s, the *Estimation and Assessment of Substance Exposure* (EASE) method was recommended for estimating exposure to notified substances. Since 1998, various simplified assessment methods have been developed, including the assessment method developed by the CRAM (7).

The principle of risk assessment using this method is based on simplified risk analyses to determine the hazardous situations associated with the handling of disinfectants and to estimate the seriousness of the potential damage and the level of exposure to each product, so that the priorities of the action plan can be determined.

The difficulty lies in gathering the data needed to define the different levels of danger on the basis of SDSs, risk phrases, labelling and exposure limit values. In our study, the SDSs for two of the 9 products were missing. In Europe, legislation requires manufacturers to provide SDSs for hazardous substances and preparations or those containing at least one substance hazardous to health or the environment (55). Similarly, although hazard labelling is a very useful piece of information, the information it contains is often incomplete and limited in number (53). Finally, the use of occupational exposure limit values to estimate toxicity levels does nothing to characterise the hazards (56).

To compensate for these shortcomings, we have taken into account elements drawn from other sources of information, such as toxicological data sheets produced by INRS or specialised databases available on the Internet for assessing the toxic risk of certain products (57).

Our assessment of the real risks took into account the respiratory and cutaneous exposure routes (as in the Rhodia method (58)), which are the two most frequent exposure routes in the workplace.

The substances used, whether pre-disinfectants or disinfectants, to which hospital staff may be exposed, belong to three main families: aldehydes, quaternary ammoniums and biguanides.

4.1 Aldehydes :

The instrumentalists in our study frequently used aldehydes, in particular glutaraldehyde and formaldehyde, to disinfect instruments, endoscopes and surfaces, without adequate means of protection.

Because of their antimicrobial effectiveness, aldehydes are widely used for terminal disinfection, disinfection of floors and surfaces, disinfection of suction systems and hemodialysis equipment, linen and bedpans...

Aldehydes are widely used for disinfecting medical instruments and equipment, in particular glutaraldehyde, which for a long time was the benchmark product for cold-soaking sterilisation of heat-sensitive equipment (in particular endoscopes). However, their use in this field is being called into question because of their ineffectiveness against non-conventional transmissible agents (prions), whose resistance to other disinfection methods they increase. The use of substitute products is currently being studied (59).

Aldehydes are formulated alone, combined with each other or over-activated by other compounds, mainly quaternary ammoniums (synergistic action).

Formaldehyde and glutaraldehyde are listed in the Hazardous Substances Data *Bank* (HSDB) as being used in certain healthcare sectors (60).

4.1.1 Glutaraldehyde :

Glutaraldehyde is used mainly for disinfecting endoscopes. It is supplied as a 2% aqueous solution and has bactericidal, virucidal, fungicidal and sporicidal properties.

The effects currently described in humans are significant irritation of the skin, trail and respiratory tract, as well as skin and respiratory allergies. No studies have demonstrated a carcinogenic, mutagenic or reprotoxic effect in humans (61,62).

In a study of healthcare workers (55), based on glutaraldehyde patch test results, their risk of being allergic was 8 times higher than that of people who did not perform this activity (prevalence of 17.6%, versus 1.9%) (63).

These factors have prompted a search for a substitute for glutaraldehyde in everyday use. Orthophthalaldehyde (OPA), a new product whose efficacy as a high-level disinfectant with a shorter use-by period has been proven in several studies, could become an interesting alternative to glutaraldehyde (64).

4.1.2 Formaldehyde :

Formaldehyde continues to be used as a high-level disinfectant in many operating theatres, even though its use for this purpose is prohibited in the United States.

developed because of its cancer-causing effects. In addition to its irritant and allergenic effects, it has been classified as a Group 1 carcinogen by the International Agency for

Research on Cancer (IARC) since June 2004, and some studies have shown an increase in nasopharyngeal cancers (65,66). In addition, its very high volatility in relation to its low boiling point (at -9°C) has earned it a risk score for inhalation ten times higher than that of glutaraldehyde under the same conditions of use. All these arguments lead us to insist on the need to replace formaldehyde in disinfection procedures for heat-sensitive and surgical equipment. Glutaraldehyde, which has no carcinogenic effect, can be offered as an alternative, subject to effective ventilation, because of its irritant and allergenic properties.

4.2 Quaternary ammoniums

These are cationic surfactants with the following properties: high washing power (detergent action), potentiation of the activity of aldehydes, but a narrow anti-bacterial spectrum (67).

The main compounds are benzalkonium chloride, cetylpyrimidium chloride, cetrinium bromide (cetrimide), didecyldimethylammonium chloride and cethexonium bromide.

They are increasingly used in healthcare settings for surface and instrument disinfection, skin antisepsis, and also in nasal and ophthalmological medicinal preparations and as a preservative in cosmetic products (68,69).

They mainly have an irritant action with a low risk of sensitisation (29,70). Quaternary ammoniums are mainly responsible for contact irritation dermatitis. Benzalkonium chloride has been frequently incriminated as a contact allergen due to numerous positive epicutaneous tests. Due to its irritant potential, a certain number of reported cases of presumed allergic contact dermatitis to benzalkonium chloride correspond to errors in the interpretation of epicutaneous tests (false positives) (71), according to Basketter and Kimber (71), it is a very rare skin sensitiser. Didecyldimethylammonium chloride, which is very irritating, and other quaternary ammoniums have only rarely been incriminated in allergic contact dermatitis.

4.3 Biguanides

The biguanides contained in certain disinfectants in combination with quaternary ammoniums are generally irritants.

Chlorhexidine, which belongs to the biguanide group, is a sensitising molecule which can cause IgE-dependent urticarial or anaphylactic reactions when used as a topical disinfectant (72). Its spraying in alcoholic solution as a biocide for surface disinfection may be responsible for occupational asthma (73).

Other biguanides may be used, and a case of allergy to polyhexamethylene biguanide has been described by Schnuch (69).

5 Prevention

5.1 Technical prevention

5.1.1 Collective prevention :

- Substitution and/or withdrawal of powerful irritants and allergens: studies are underway to replace glutaraldehyde in the disinfection of flexible endoscopes (buffered peracetic acid, chlorine agents) (74,75). However, the antimicrobial efficacy of these disinfectants suggests toxicity in humans, and care must be taken to avoid "displacing" the risk; for example, the replacement of formaldehyde by glutaraldehyde has led to an increase in the number of cases of sensitisation to glutaraldehyde at the same time as a decrease in cases of sensitisation to formaldehyde;

- Disinfection should be limited to the premises where it is needed, avoiding the use of sprays;

- Use autoclavable equipment as often as possible;

- Disinfection by cold soaking reserved exclusively for heat-sensitive equipment (flexible endoscopes, invasive ultrasound probes); sealed endoscope washers, with systematic drying cycle;

- Automation using disinfectant in a closed circuit; for manual disinfection, the containers must be covered;

- Ventilation of the work area, capture of disinfectants at source and discharge outside the area;

\-   Informing staff about the health risks of products, complying with conditions of use and reading labels.

5.1.2 Individual prevention :

Individual prevention is based on wearing gloves:

\-   PVC (or vinyl) or nitrile gloves are preferable to latex, which can cause allergies;

\-   latex, vinyl and polyethylene medical gloves offer good protection against glutaraldehyde (permeation time greater than 60 minutes) (76). However, butyl rubber gloves are more effective (permeation time greater than 4 hours for glutaraldehyde) (77).

On the other hand, isopropyl and ethyl alcohols penetrate latex and vinyl gloves rapidly (permeation time less than 10 minutes for isopropyl alcohol) and deteriorate them (76).

Depending on the activity, we also recommend wearing protective clothing and personal protective equipment such as a waterproof apron, goggles or a face shield, a respiratory protection mask adapted to the type of product and boots.

5.2 Medical prevention :

As with all prevention of contact dermatitis on the hands, washing with mild cleaning products and frequent and regular application of emollients are necessary. Antiseptic hand washing should be reserved for stains requiring it.

During the annual medical check-up, the interviewer looks for oculonasal, bronchial and/or cutaneous symptoms at the same time as the disinfection operations.

In allergic patients, it is essential to avoid contact with the allergen. This involves identifying all professional and domestic sources of the allergen.

6   Repair :

A number of occupational dermatoses caused by disinfectants and antiseptics are included in the list of compensable occupational diseases (Table X).

Table XI: Compensable occupational skin diseases

Table MP	Designation of dermatological diseases	Agents involved
n° 28: formic aldehyde and its polymers	Subacute or chronic eczematiform dermatitis.	Formaldehyde, its solutions (formaldehyde) and its polymers
n° 59: Other agents responsible for eczematiform dermatoses of allergic mechanism	Recurrent eczematiform lesions after new exposure to the risk or confirmed by a positive epicutaneous test for the product handled.	Quaternary ammoniums and their salts, especially in cationic detergents

5 CONCLUSION

Disinfectants are chemical formulations combining a variety of antimicrobial agents with excipients, cleaning agents and adjuvants. Their widespread use, due to the intensification of anti-infectious measures, particularly in healthcare departments, is the source of many occupational dermatoses, especially irritant and/or allergic contact dermatitis.

The aims of this study were to detect occupational dermatitis in instrument technicians, to assess the chemical risk associated with the use of disinfectants in operating theatres, and to propose appropriate preventive measures.

Our study was a descriptive cross-sectional study conducted in the operating theatre of the CHU Habib Bourguiba and the gynaecology theatre of the CHU Hedi Chaker in Sfax, Tunisia, over a period of 2 months. The population studied consisted of instrumentalists assigned to these operating theatres and performing the disinfection task. Data was collected using a pre-established form. The form included socio-demographic and occupational characteristics, medical history (particularly dermatological), and clinical data from the interview and dermatological examination to detect any dermatosis. The occupational origin of the dermatosis was selected on the basis of the Mathias criteria. We completed our study with an assessment of the chemical risk associated with the use of disinfectants in operating theatres, using an occupational risk assessment guide drawn up by the CRAM.

Forty-five instrumentalists took part in the survey, giving a participation rate of 71.4%. The mean age of the study population was 39.7 years. More than half of the participants (60%) were female, with a sex ratio of 0.66. The study population was made up of 64% senior operating theatre technicians and 36% nurses, with an average working life of 14.2 years. Dermatological antecedents were noted in 10 cases. Most of these were irritant dermatitis (5 cases). A history of personal atopy was reported by 15.7% of instrumentalists. A history of allergic rhinitis was noted in 46.7% of cases, asthma in 11.1% and respiratory irritation in 1 case. By carrying out a detailed interview and clinical examination of lesions present on the day of the survey, we identified 8 new cases of contact dermatitis of the DIC (5 cases), DAC (1 case) and urticaria (2 cases) type. According to Mathias' criteria, the diagnosis of occupational dermatosis was retained in 31.1% of instrumentalists. Numerous studies in the literature confirmed the high risk of occupational dermatoses in the healthcare sector, with a prevalence of around 20-30%. In our study, these dermatoses included irritant contact dermatitis (10 cases), allergic contact dermatitis (2 cases) and urticaria (2 cases). This result was consistent with several international studies which had shown that ICD is more common than CDD in healthcare workers. This frequency of ICD in this sector of activity, and particularly among the instrumentalists in our study, can be explained by the fact that these employees regularly used disinfectant products during disinfection procedures. Most of these products are highly irritant and are therefore probably largely responsible for the appearance of irritative lesions in these subjects. The contact urticaria found in 2 cases in our population was very probably linked to an allergy to the latex proteins contained in the gloves. In Higgins' study, skin allergy to latex gloves accounted for 13% of occupational dermatitis in healthcare workers. However, certain antiseptics or disinfectants can also cause contact urticaria (chlorhexidine, polyvidone iodine, formaldehyde, chloramine). With regard to extracutaneous symptoms associated with the use of disinfectants, signs of rhinitis were found in 40% of instrumentalists. Symptoms suggestive of a respiratory gene related to the handling of disinfectants were found in 7 instrumentalists. Signs of conjunctivitis were reported by 9 instrumentalists (20%). Along with latex, disinfectants used in medical environments are the most frequent causes of occupational asthma.

The assessment of the chemical risk associated with the use of disinfectants consisted of an inventory of the disinfectant products used, which were mainly based on quaternary ammoniums, glutaraldehyde, formaldehyde and biguanides. In the case of glutaraldehyde, the effects currently described in humans are significant irritation of the skin, the respiratory tract and the respiratory tract, as well as skin and respiratory allergies. No studies have demonstrated a carcinogenic, mutagenic or reprotoxic effect in humans. Formaldehyde, used as a high-level disinfectant in many operating theatres, has a cancerogenic effect in addition to its irritant and allergenic effects. As for quaternary ammoniums and biguanides, they mainly have an irritant action with a low risk of sensitisation. Applying the occupational risk assessment guide therefore enabled us to identify the hazardous situations associated with each disinfectant product, to estimate for each hazardous situation the severity of the potential damage and the frequency of exposure of employees to the hazards, and to conclude on the priority for action based on these last two parameters in order to propose preventive measures adapted to each risk.

Following this assessment, technical, organisational and educational preventive measures will be the only alternative for controlling the chemical risk in this sector. Such measures require the involvement of operators, management, administration, occupational health physicians and hygiene technicians, and will help to control the risk and promote the health of workers in this sector.

6 REFERENCES

1. SFHH. Liste positive desinfectants June 2009. 2009;

2. Crepy M. Dermatoses professionnelles aux antiseptiques et desinfectants. Doc pour le medecin du Trav. 2001;85:83-90.

3. Crepy MN. Occupational dermatoses caused by detergents. Doc pour le Medecin du Trav. 2005;375-84.

4. Billast N, Duffet AM DC. Recommendations for good practice in the use of disinfectants and antiseptics in hospitals. C-CLIN Paris-Nord. 2000;19-85.

5. Nosbaum A, Nicolas JF, Vocanson M, Rozieres A, Berard F. Allergic and irritant contact dermatitis. Sci direct. Elsevier Masson SAS; 2010;71(3):4.

6. Mathias CG. Contact dermatitis and workers' compensation: criteria for establishing occupational causation and aggravation. J Am Acad Dermatol. 1989 May;20(5 Pt 1):842-8.

7. Guide d'évaluation des risques professionals CRAM.

8. Mathias CG. Contact dermatitis from use or misuse of soaps, detergents, and cleansers in the workplace. Occup Med. 1(2):205-18.

9. Hecht G, Subra I, Gerber JM, Hubert G. Exposure to chemicals in the food industry. 1999;

10. Jungbauer FHW, van der Vleuten P, Groothoff JW, Coenraads PJ. Irritant hand dermatitis: severity of disease, occupational exposure to skin irritants and preventive measures 5 years after initial diagnosis. Contact Dermatitis. 2004 Apr;50(4):245-51.

11. Kostner L, Anzengruber F, Guillod C, Recher M, Schmid-Grendelmeier P, Navarini AA. Allergic contact dermatitis. Immunol Allergy Clin North Am. 2017;37(1):141- 52.

12. Stingeni L, Lapomarda V, Lisi P. Occupational hand dermatitis in hospital environments. Contact Dermatitis. 1995 Sep;33(3):172-6.

13. Garon-Michel N, Paul M, Lodde B, Roguedas-Contios AM, Misery L. Consultation specialisee de dermatologie professionnelle : bilan de cinq ans d'activite. Place de l'atopie.

Ann Dermatol Venereol. 2010;137(11):681-7.

14. Susceptibility to and incidence of hand dermatitis in a cohort of apprentice hairdressers and nurses. | Base documentaire | BDSP [Internet]. [cited 2019 Jan 22]. Available from: http://www.bdsp.ehesp.fr

15. Turner S, Carder M, Van Tongeren M, McNamee R, Lines S, Hussey L, et al. The incidence of occupational skin disease as reported to the Health and Occupation Reporting (THOR) network between 2002 and 2005. Br J Dermatol. 2007;157(4):713- 22.

16. Mahler V, Bruckner T, Schmidt A, Diepgen TL. Occupational contact dermatitis in health care workers. Contact Dermatitis. John Wiley & Sons, Ltd (10.1111); 2008 Jun 28;50(3):158-9.

17. Ibler KS, Jemec GBE, Flyvholm M-A, Diepgen TL, Jensen A, Agner T. Hand eczema: prevalence and risk factors of hand eczema in a population of 2274 healthcare workers. Contact Dermatitis. 2012 Oct;67(4):200-7.

18. Flyvholm M-A, Bach B, Rose M, Jepsen KF. Self-reported hand eczema in a hospital population. Contact Dermatitis. 2007 Aug;57(2):110 -5.

19. IVDK - Comite Surveillance Evaluation Scientifique des Allergies de Contact - Adjocom [Internet]. [cited 2019 Jan 22]. Available from: https://adjocom.com/content/638-ivdk-allergie-contact

20. Diepgen TL, Coenraads PJ. The epidemiology of occupational contact dermatitis. Int Arch Occup Environ Health. 1999 Nov;72(8):496-506.

21. Holness DL, Mace SR. Results of evaluating health care workers with prick and patch testing. Am J Contact Dermat. 2001 Jun;12(2):88-92.

22. Larese Filon F, Bochdanovits L, Capuzzo C, Cerchi R, Rui F. Ten-year incidence of natural rubber latex sensitization and symptoms in a prospective cohort of health care workers using non-powdered latex gloves 2000-2009. Int Arch Occup Environ Health. 2014 Jul 23;87(5):463-9.

23. Nettis E, Colanardi MC, Soccio AL, Ferrannini A, Tursi A. Occupational irritant and allergic contact dermatitis among healthcare workers. Contact Dermatitis. 2002 Feb;46(2):101-7.

24. Misery L, Paul M, Lodde B. Occupational dermatoses induced by de A propos de 50 patients d'une consultation de dermatologie professionnelle. 2009;437-45.

25. Higgins CL, Palmer AM, Cahill JL, Nixon RL. Occupational skin disease among Australian healthcare workers: a retrospective analysis from an occupational dermatology clinic, 1993-2014. Contact Dermatitis. 2016;75(4):213-22.

26. Pesonen M, Jolanki R, Larese Filon F, Wilkinson M, Kr^cisz B, Kiec-Swierczynska M, et al. Patch test results of the European baseline series among patients with occupational contact dermatitis across Europe - analyses of the European Surveillance System on Contact Allergy network, 2002-2010. Contact Dermatitis. 2015 Mar;72(3):154-63.

27. Kucenic MJ, Belsito D V. Occupational allergic contact dermatitis is more prevalent than irritant contact dermatitis: a 5-year study. J Am Acad Dermatol. 2002 May;46(5):695-9.

28. Warshaw EM, Schram SE, Maibach HI, Belsito D V, Marks JG, Fowler JF, et al. Occupation-related contact dermatitis in North American health care workers referred for patch testing: cross-sectional data, 1998 to 2004. Dermat contact, atopic, Occup drug. 19(5):261-74.

29. Schnuch A, Uter W, Geier J, Frosch PJ, Rustemeyer T. Contact allergies in healthcare workers. Results from the IVDK. Acta Derm Venereol. 1998;78(5):358 -63.

30. Dickel H, Kuss O, Schmidt A, Kretz J, Diepgen TL. Importance of Irritant Contact Dermatitis in Occupational Skin Disease. Am J Clin Dermatol. 2002;3(4):283-9.

31. Kampf G, Ennen J. Regular use of a hand cream can attenuate skin dryness and roughness caused by frequent hand washing. BMC Dermatol. 2006 Feb 13;6(1):1.

32. Lim YL, Goon A. Occupational skin diseases in Singapore 2003-2004: an epidemiologic update. Contact Dermatitis. 2007 Mar;56(3):157-9.

33. Ebo DG, Stevens WJ, Bridts CH, Matthieu L. Contact allergic dermatitis and lifethreatening anaphylaxis to chlorhexidine. J Allergy Clin Immunol. 1998 Jan;101(1):128-9.

34. Autegarden JE, Pecquet C, Huet S, Bayrou O, Leynadier F. Anaphylactic shock after application of chlorhexidine to unbroken skin. Contact Dermatitis. 1999 Apr;40(4):215.

35. Okano M, Nomura M, Hata S, Okada N, Sato K, Kitano Y, et al. Anaphylactic symptoms due to chlorhexidine gluconate. Arch Dermatol. 1989 Jan;125(1):50-2.

36. AMEILLE J. C, A R. Occupational asthma in France. Assessment of 3 years of operation of the national observatory of occupational asthma (ONAP). Arch des Mal Prof. 2000;

37. Current asthma: Estimated prevalence by industry and sex, U.S. working adults aged >18 years, NHIS 2004-2011 [Internet]. [cited 2019 Jan 24]. Available from: https://wwwn.cdc.gov/eworld/Data/Current_asthma_Estimated_prevalence_by_industr y_and_sex_US_working_adults_aged_18_years_NHIS

38. Quinn MM, Henneberger PK, Braun B, Delclos GL, Fagan K, Huang V, et al. Cleaning and disinfecting environmental surfaces in health care: Toward an integrated framework for infection and occupational illness prevention. Am J Infect Control. Mosby; 2015 May 1;43(5):424-34.

39. Arif AA, Delclos GL. Association between cleaning-related chemicals and work- related asthma and asthma symptoms among healthcare professionals. Occup Env Med. BMJ Publishing Group Ltd; 2012 Jan 1;69(1):35-40.

40. Rosenman KD. Cleaning Products-related Asthma. Clin Pulm Med. Clinical Pulmonary Medicine; 2006 Jul 1;13(4):221-8.

41. Delclos GL, Gimeno D, Arif AA, Benavides FG, Zock J-P. Occupational Exposures and Asthma in Health-Care Workers: Comparison of Self-Reports With a Workplace-Specific Job Exposure Matrix. Am J Epidemiol. 2008 Dec 16;169(5):581-7.

42. Saito R, Virji MA, Henneberger PK, Humann MJ, LeBouf RF, Stanton ML, et al. Characterization of cleaning and disinfecting tasks and product use among hospital

occupations. Am J Ind Med. John Wiley & Sons, Ltd; 2015 Jan 1;58(1):101-11.

43. Beckett WS, Box MPH. Revised Protocol: Criteria for Designating Substances as Occupational Asthmagens on the AOEC List of Exposure Codes.

44. Bernstein JA, Stauder T, Bernstein DI, Bernstein IL. A combined respiratory and cutaneous hypersensitivity syndrome induced by work exposure to quaternary amines. J Allergy Clin Immunol. 1994 Aug;94(2 Pt 1):257-9.

45. Corrado OJ, Osman J, Davies RJ. Asthma and rhinitis after exposure to glutaraldehyde in endoscopy units. Hum Toxicol. 1986 Sep;5(5):325-8.

46. Quirce S, Gomez M, Bombrn C, Sastre J. Glutaraldehyde-induced asthma. Allergy. 1999 Oct;54(10):1121-2.

47. Kramps JA, van Toorenenbergen AW, Vooren PH, Dijkman JH. Occupational asthma due to inhalation of chloramine-T. II. Demonstration of specific IgE antibodies. Int Arch Allergy Appl Immunol. 1981;64(4):428-38.

48. Jacson F, Beaudouin E, Hotton J, Moneret-Vautrin DA. Allergie au formol, latex et oxy de d'ethylene : triple allergie professionnelle chez une infirmiere. Rev Francaise d' Allergologie d'Immunologie Clin. Elsevier Masson; 1991 Jan 1;31(1):41-3.

49. Dooms-Goossens A, Gevers D, Mertens A, Vanderheyden D. Allergic contact urticaria due to chloramine. Contact Dermatitis. 1983 Jul;9(4):319-20.

50. Ong TH, Tan KL, Lee HS, Eng P. A case report of occupational asthma due to gluteraldehyde exposure. Ann Acad Med Singapore. 2004 Mar;33(2):275-8.

51. Hendrick DJ, Lane DJ. Occupational formalin asthma. Br J Ind Med. 1977 Feb;34(1):11-8.

52. Burge PS, Richardson MN. Occupational asthma due to indirect exposure to lauryl dimethyl benzyl ammonium chloride used in a floor cleaner. Thorax. 1994 Aug;49(8):842-3.

53. Institut national de la sante et de la recherche medicale (INSERM). Risque chimique septembre 2002 [Internet]. [cited 2019 Jan 24]. Available from: https://www.inserm.fr

54. Vincent R. Methodologie d' évaluation simplifiee du risque chimique. Hygiene securite du Trav - Cah notes Doc. 2005;39-62.

55. Pilliere F, Triolet J RM. La fiche de donnee de securite . Cah notes Doc - Hygiene securite du Trav. 1998;2089:173.

56. Vincent R, Bonthoux F. Hierarchisation des " risques potentiels ". 2000;

57. TOXNET [Internet]. [cited 2019 Jan 24]. Available from: https://toxnet.nlm.nih.gov/

58. R. Persoons, L. Dumas, M. Stoklov AM. Development of a new chemical risk assessment method: application in hospital laboratories. Arch Mal Prof Env. 2005;326-34.

59. R, AUDOUIN O, K. Is glutaraldehyde essential for disinfecting medical equipment? Study of alternative solutions and organisation of endoscope disinfection in a 21st century hospital. , 2000, 47 p. Fac medecine, Cochin Port-Royal, Memoire pour l'obtention du diplome d'etudes specialisees en Medecine du Travail. 2000;47.

60. Hazardous Substances Data Bank (HSDB) [Internet]. [cited 2019 Jan 24]. Available from: https://toxnet.nlm.nih.gov/cgi-bin/sis/htmlgen?HSDB

61. TESTUD F. Toxicologie medicale professionnelle et environnementale. Eska, Environmental Medicine. 2012;815.

62. Glutaraldehyde. Fiche toxicologique n°171. INRS. 2018;1-10.

63. Shaffer MP, Belsito D V. Allergic contact dermatitis from glutaraldehyde in healthcare workers. Contact Dermatitis. 2000 Sep;43(3):150 -6.

64. Rutala WA, Weber DJ. Disinfection of endoscopes: review of new chemical sterilants used for high-level disinfection. Infect Control Hosp Epidemiol. 1999 Jan 2;20(1):69- 76.

65. Institut National de Recherche et de Securite. Le formaldehyde. Point des connaissances ; ED : 5032.

66. Hauptmann M, Lubin JH, Stewart PA, Hayes RB, Blair A. Mortality from Solid Cancers among Workers in Formaldehyde Industries. Am J Epidemiol. 2004 Jun 15;159(12):1117-30.

67. CHABEAU G. Les decontaminants de surface : faut-il s'en laver les mains ? 12 e cours

de dermato-allergologie. Strasbourg, GERDA. 1991. p. 243-51.

68. Cusano F, Luciano S. Contact allergy to benzalkonium chloride and glutaraldehyde in a dental nurse. Contact Dermatitis. 1993 Feb;28(2):127.

69. Schnuch A, Geier J, Brasch J, Fuchs T, Pirker C, Schulze-Dirks A, et al. Polyhexamethylenebiguanide: a relevant contact allergen? Contact Dermatitis. 2000 May;42(5):302-3.

70. Engebretsen KA, Hald M, Johansen JD, Thyssen JP. Allergic contact dermatitis caused by an antiseptic containing cetrimide. Contact Dermatitis. 2015 Jan;72(1):60-1.

71. Basketter DA, Kimber I. Skin sensitization, false positives and false negatives: experience with guinea pig assays. J Appl Toxicol. 2010 Jul 28;30(5):381-6.

72. Ohtoshi T, Yamauchi N, Tadokoro K, Miyachi S, Suzuki S, Miyamoto T, et al. IgE antibody-mediated shock reaction caused by topical application of chlorhexidine. Clin Allergy. 1986 Mar;16(2):155-61.

73. Waclawski ER, McAlpine LG, Thomson NC. Occupational asthma in nurses caused by chlorhexidine and alcohol aerosols. BMJ. 1989 Apr 8;298(6678):929-30.

74. DOMART M, PINEAU J HE. CLIN/HEGP working group. Evaluation of different automatic disinfection procedures for flexible endoscopes. Personal communication.

75. O'DONOVAN M. Glutaraldehyde hazards: What is the alternative? The Safety and Health Practitioner. 1996;14:73-5.

76. Mellstrom GA, Lindberg M, Boman A. Permeation and destructive effects of disinfectants on protective gloves. Contact Dermatitis. 1992 Mar;26(3):163-70.

77. Lehman PA, Franz TJ, Guin JD. Penetration of glutaraldehyde through glove material: Tactylon versus natural rubber latex. Contact Dermatitis. 1994 Mar;30(3):176-7.

Survey form

Socio-professional characteristics

- Age : /-/-/ years

- Sex : M ☐   F ☐

- Block :

- Grade: senior technician ☐ nurse ☐

- Professional experience: / / years   / years

- Number of hours worked per day: /--/ h

- Working hours: fixed: morning ☐ afternoon ☐ night ☐

Variable: morning ☐ afternoon ☐ night ☐

- Leisure activities :

Pathological antecedents

- Personal atopy yes ☐   no ☐ type :

- Familial atopy: yes ☐   no ☐ type:

- Respiratory history: rhinitis ☐ asthma ☐

- Dermatological history: urticaria ☐ eczema ☐ irritant dermatitis ☐ other :

- Other antecedents:

Professional survey

- What products do you use to disinfect operating instruments and operating theatres?

- **How many times a day do you disinfect instruments? /-/**

What type of gloves do you use for disinfection?

clean gloves ☐ latex ☐ rubber ☐   PVC ☐

Are these gloves suitable (long-sleeved gloves) yes ☐ no ☐

- **Do you wear protective goggles when disinfecting? yes ☐ no ☐**

- **Do you wear masks during disinfection? yes ☐   no ☐**

- **Are you aware of the procedures and rules for using disinfectants?**

yes ☐ no ☐

- **Are you aware of the health risks associated with disinfectants?**

yes ☐ no ☐

<u>Respiratory effects</u>

- **Have you consulted a doctor about rhinitis and/or asthma?**

Yes ☐ No ☐ If yes, since when? / --- /

- **Do you have any of the following signs?**

Nasal pruritus ☐ sneezing ☐   Nasal obstruction ☐

rhinorrhea ☐ chronic cough ☐   dyspnea ☐ oppression

thoracic ☐

- **Are these signs improved during leave? yes ☐   no ☐**

<u>Skin effects</u>

- **Have you consulted a doctor about skin lesions?**

yes ☐ **no** ☐ **If yes, since when** //?

What type? irritant dermatitis ☐ **contact eczema** ☐ **urticaria** ☐

Others :

- **Did you develop skin lesions on your hands during your work? yes** ☐ **no** ☐

- **Onset/recruitment :**

- **If so, these lesions are :**

Squamous erythematous ☐ **Vesicular erythematous** ☐ **Papulo erythematous** ☐

contours well limited to the contact area ☐ **flakes extending beyond the contact area** ☐

burning sensation ☐ **oozing pruritus** ☐

fleeting ☐

- **are they improved during leave?**

yes ☐ **no** ☐

- **Have you had these skin lesions investigated?**

yes ☐ **no** ☐

Type: patch test ☐ prick test ☐ specific tests (open test; roat test; use test) ☐

CBC ☐   Total IgE ☐   Specific IgE ☐

- **Treatment received :**

- **Development time :**

- **Evolution :**

Persistence ☐ **Recovery** ☐   **Recidivism** ☐

■   **Behaviour in the event of a positive test:**

Refer to dermatology consultation: no ☐ **yes** ☐ **Declaration MP: no** ☐ **yes** ☐ tab.e n°

Aptitude: same workstation ☐ Professional reclassification ☐ Workstation adjustment ☐

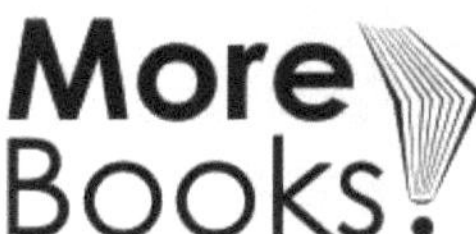

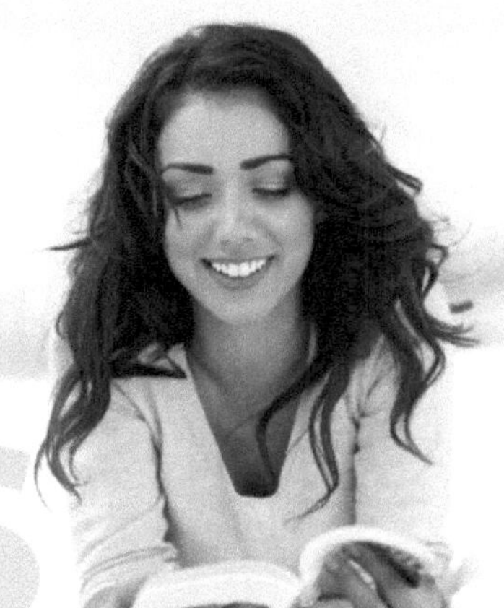

yes

I want morebooks!

Buy your books fast and straightforward online - at one of world's fastest growing online book stores! Environmentally sound due to Print-on-Demand technologies.

Buy your books online at
www.morebooks.shop

Kaufen Sie Ihre Bücher schnell und unkompliziert online – auf einer der am schnellsten wachsenden Buchhandelsplattformen weltweit! Dank Print-On-Demand umwelt- und ressourcenschonend produzi ert.

Bücher schneller online kaufen
www.morebooks.shop

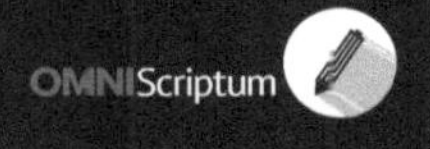

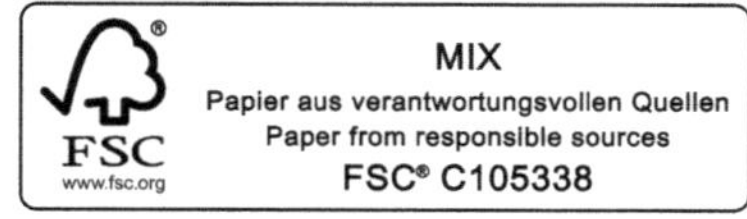

Printed by Books on Demand GmbH, Norderstedt / Germany